How to
TIE A
HEADSCARF

———

30 simple, modern styles

ALICE TATE

Abrams Image, New York

CONTENTS

INTRODUCTION

From the functional to the chic, the headscarf is the ultimate accessory. Whatever print or style you choose, scarves can be worn in so many ways to create infinite different looks, from vintage inspired to contemporary, and are great for all hairstyles.

The 30 styles in this book have been carefully curated to make sure you are covered in the most beautiful ways whatever the occasion—vacations, office days, nights out, beach trips, festivals, bad hair days, and everything in between.

BASIC FOLDS

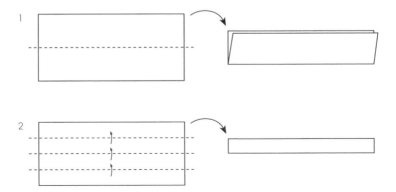

HEADSCARF BASICS

Fabric types that work well: silk, viscose, chiffon, cotton, and jersey.

Two basic headscarf shapes you need: 1 square scarf—at least
20 x 20 inches (50 cm x 50 cm), though 35 x 35 inches (90 cm
x 90 cm) is the most versatile size.
*Other square scarves used here are 24 x 24 inches (60 cm x 60 cm)
and 28 x 28 inches (70 cm x 70 cm).*

1 rectangular scarf—at least 20 x 67 inches (50 cm x 170 cm).
*Other rectangular scarves used here are 24 x 67 inches (60 cm
x 170 cm), 28 x 67 inches (70 cm x 170 cm), 28 x 70 inches (70 cm
x 180 cm), 28 x 75 inches (70 cm x 190 cm), and 35 x 70 inches
(90 cm x 180 cm). A long, thin rectangular scarf is also useful—we've
used one here that is 8 x 75 inches (20 cm x 190 cm).*

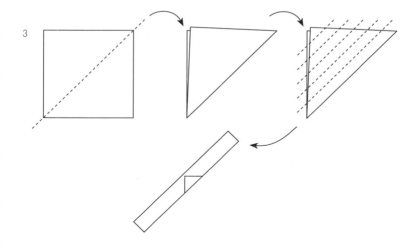

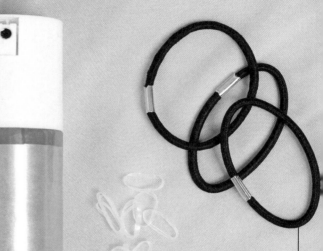

Elastics/
hair bands

Hair spray

Hair doughnut
(for maximum volume
on topknot)

Bobby pins

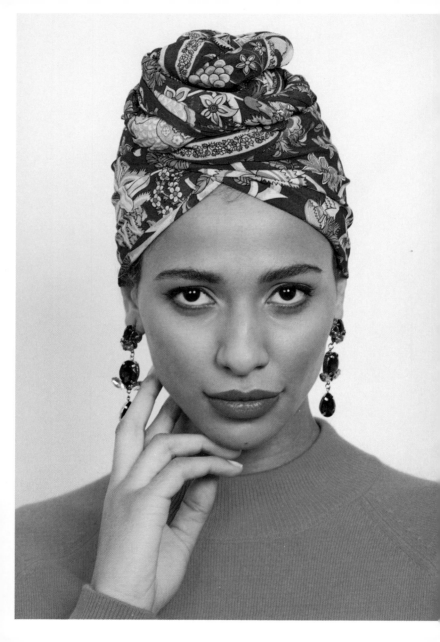

1

The KNOTTED WRAP

1: The
KNOTTED
WRAP

An easy-to-master style that
works great with braids.
Pair with sunnies, earrings,
and a bold lip to add a touch
of glamour.

We used a 28 x 75-inch
(70 x 190-cm) scarf to create
this look.

Tie your hair into a tight
topknot.

Fold a long, rectangular
scarf in half lengthwise.

Position the folded edge
of the scarf at the base of
your head, just above the
nape of your neck (1).

Tightly pull the rest of the
fabric over your head
to the center of your
forehead (2).

Separate the two ends
of the scarf and twist
together until they
resemble a rope (3).

As you do so, start
wrapping this rope into
a bun at the top of your
head. When you reach the
end, tuck the loose ends
under the bun to secure
(4). Pin in place to keep
it secure.

For the finishing touch,
add earrings to bring the
whole look together.

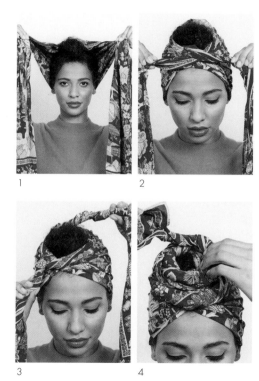

1   2

3   4

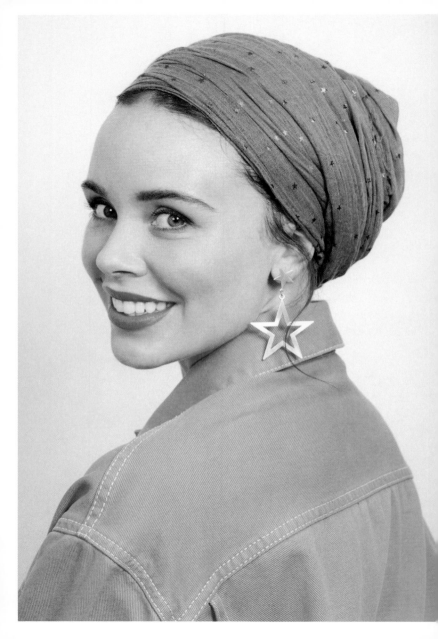

2

The TUCK-AWAY WRAP

2: The
TUCK-AWAY
WRAP

A wrapped up, sophisticated style that works for everyone and is best done with a large, rectangular scarf. Add a statement lip, specs, or earrings for a polished finish.

We used a 35 x 70-inch (90 x 180-cm) scarf to create this look.

Using a long scarf, position one of the long edges at the front of your head, along the hairline.

Take the ends over your ears and cross over at the back of your neck (1).

Wrap one end of the fabric (folded flat) around your head, secure in place (2), then wrap the other side around your head, starting slightly farther back to add a little height (3).

Tuck the end of the fabric underneath to secure in place (4).

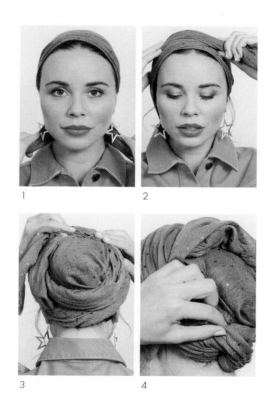

1

2

3

4

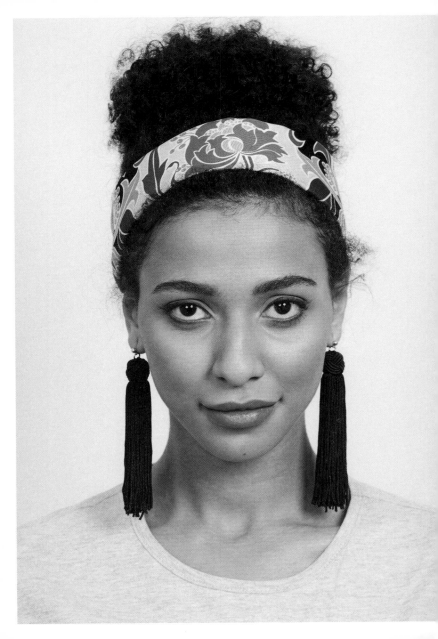

3

The HEADBAND

3: The HEADBAND

A versatile style that transforms a simple updo into a more finished look. Works best with a long, thin strip scarf. Looks great with statement earrings.

We used a 35-inch (90-cm) square scarf to create this look.

Tie hair up into a high ponytail or bun.

Using a thin, long scarf or a scarf folded into a neat long strip, wrap the fabric tightly around the head (1), securing at the nape of the neck with a knot (2).

Tuck the ends of the fabric underneath to neaten and secure in place (3).

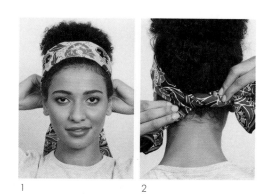

1

2

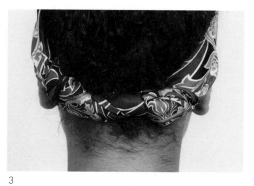

3

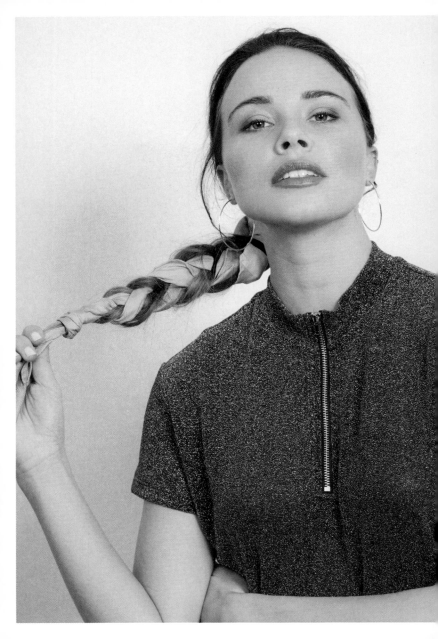

4

The RIBBON BRAID

4: The
RIBBON
BRAID

Transform a simple braid into a sartorial statement by weaving in a printed headscarf. Easy-peasy wow factor.

We used a 28-inch (70-cm) square scarf to create this look.

Tie the hair into a low ponytail and tie the scarf around the elastic to cover the band (1).

Separate the hair into three strands as you would a braid, adding the two ends of the scarf into the outer sections (2).

Braid the hair loosely, incorporating the fabric as you go (3).

When you get to the end, either tie with an elastic (4), or, if there is enough of the fabric left, you can wrap the ends of the scarf around the braid to secure and fasten into a bow.

Pull out strands and wispy bits to give a more relaxed and effortless look.

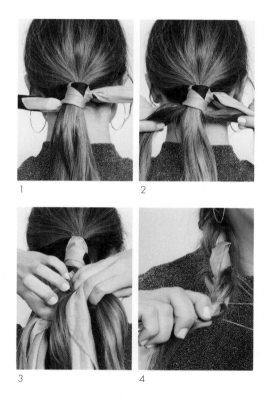

1

2

3

4

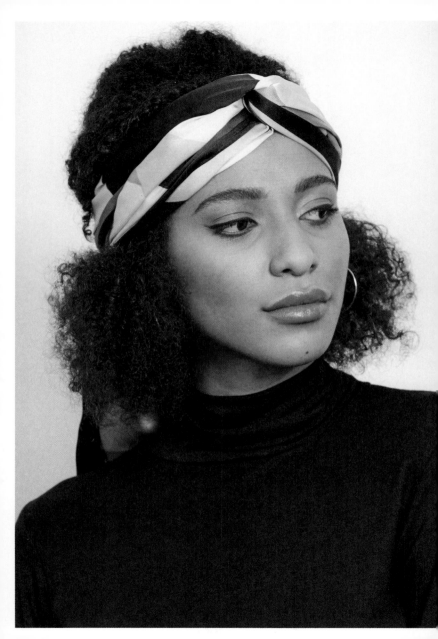

5

The PARISIAN TWIST

5: The PARISIAN TWIST

Add a touch of Parisian chic to your ensemble with this relaxed, twisted band style. This also works well with a low, loose ponytail.

We used a 28 x 70-inch (70 x 180-cm) scarf to create this look.

Fold a rectangular scarf to create a long band or use a long, thin scarf for this look.

With the hair down or in a low, relaxed ponytail, take the scarf to the nape of the neck.

Bring both ends up, over the ears, until they cross at the top of the head (1).

Then twist at the forehead until they are, once again, in line with the band (2 & 3).

Bring the ends back down, past the ears, to knot securely at the back (4 & 5).

Pull out any loose, wispy strands to give a more relaxed finish.

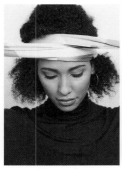

1

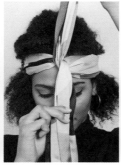

2

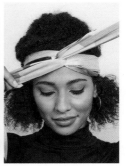

3

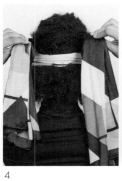

4

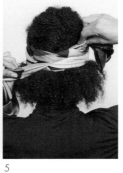

5

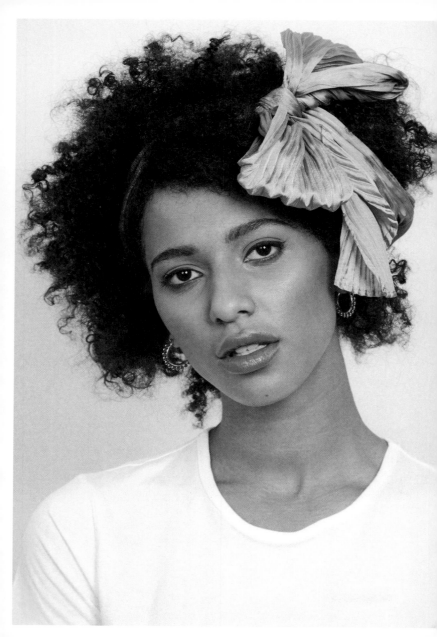

6

The BOHO BOW

6: The
BOHO BOW

Transform a basic updo into a cool, hippie look with this relaxed boho bow—an easy outfit finisher. Works well with wispy bangs.

We used a 8 x 75-inch (20 x 190-cm) scarf to create this look.

Tie the hair into a comfortable ponytail or low bun if you have long hair, or leave down.

Pull out the front strands or bangs to give a more relaxed look.

Take a long, thin scarf to the back of the neck (1).

Tie both ends into a comfortable bow at the front (2).

Pull the ends to make the bow as large or as small as you wish, and position slightly to the side (3).

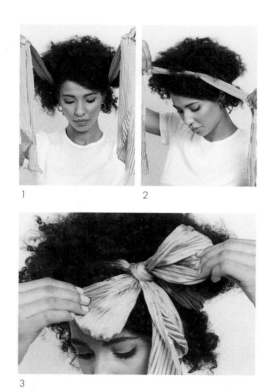

1

2

3

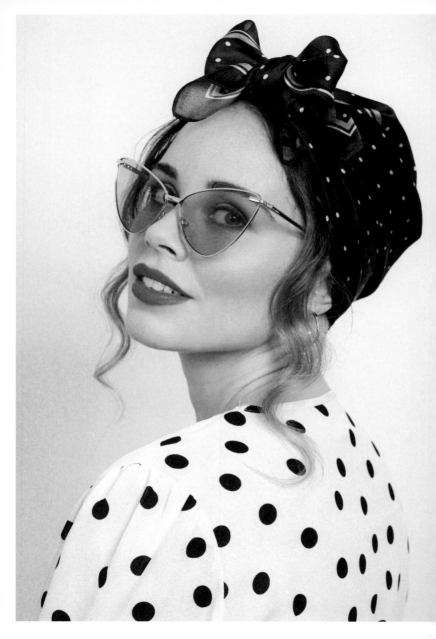

7

The FORTIES WRAP

7: The
FORTIES WRAP

Channel times gone by with this retro forties wrap—an easy-to-master style that makes the perfect accessory for a vintage look.

We used a 28-inch (70-cm) square scarf to create this look.

With hair tied up at the back of the head, fold a square scarf into a triangle and place the fold at the nape of the neck. The triangle should be resting on the forehead (1).

Draw the two ends of the fabric up over your ears to meet at the top, and tie tightly (2), trapping the point underneath so the fabric covers the back and crown of the head.

Tie the ends of the fabric, including the point, into a bow, and pull out any loose strands to create a more relaxed look.

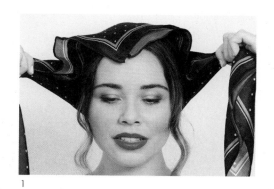

1

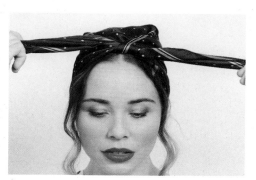

2

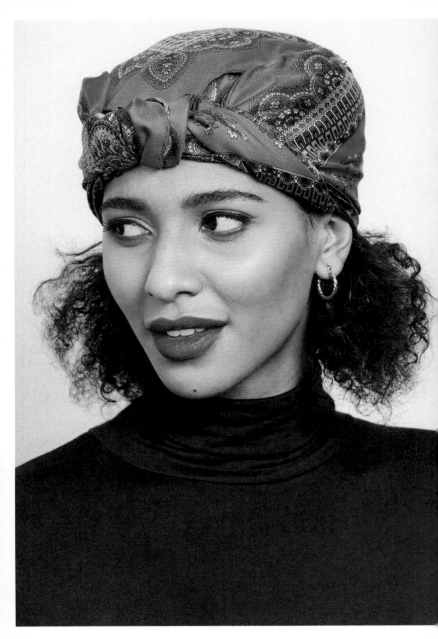

8

The MESSY HAIR HIDEAWAY

8: The
MESSY HAIR
HIDEAWAY

Cover a million sins—bad hair days, dirty roots, and flyaways—with this statement headscarf that works well with your hair up or down.

We used a 35-inch (90-cm) square scarf to create this look.

With hair left loose, fold a large, square scarf into a triangle and take the fold to the base of the head (1).

Pull both layers of the point over the head and both ends up, past the ears, to meet at the top.

Tie all ends into a knot so the scarf sits securely on the head (2).

Once in place, tuck the ends of the scarf under the front so they're hidden, and let the last layer you tuck under cover the knot (3 & 4).

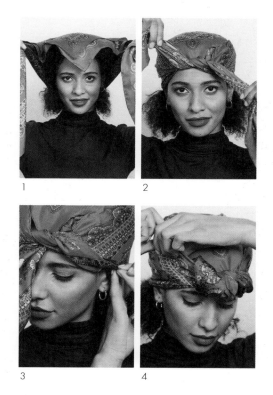

1

2

3

4

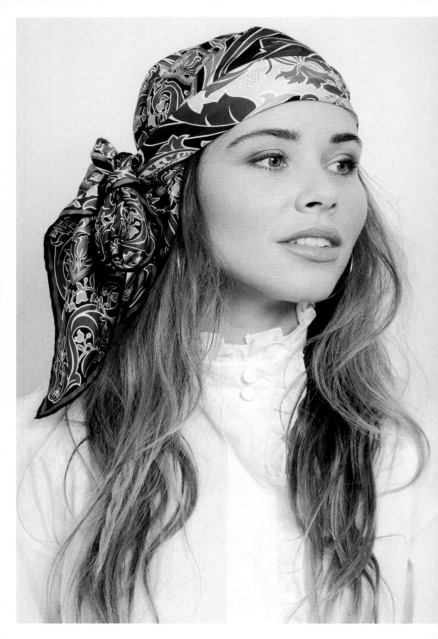

9

The PIRATE SCARF

9: The PIRATE SCARF

A simple, bohemian-chic style that adds a touch of glamour to any outfit. Works best with the hair left loose—a great trick for hiding unwashed roots.

We used a 35-inch (90-cm) square scarf to create this look.

With the hair left loose, take a large, square scarf and fold it into a triangle.

Pull the scarf over your head so that the long point of the scarf is either to the left or right of your head (1 & 2).

Tie the ends together, trapping the fabric and the point underneath (3).

Arrange as feels and looks comfortable, then tie the ends into a bow (4).

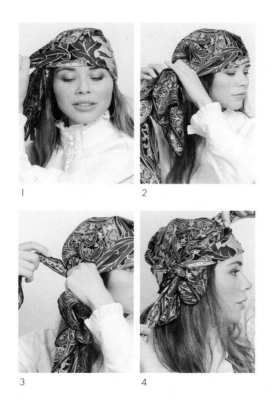

1

2

3

4

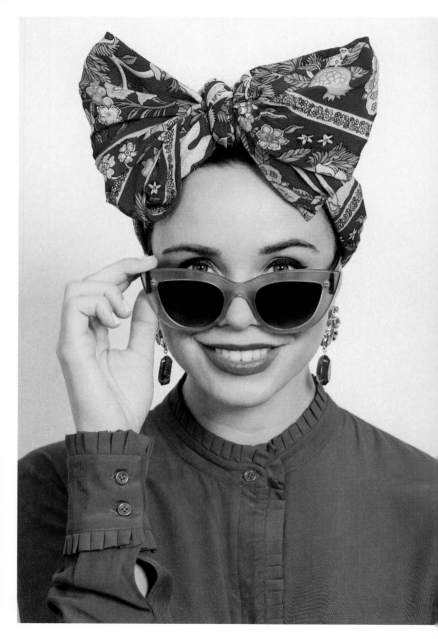

10

The STATEMENT BOW

10: The STATEMENT BOW

Go big and go bold with this statement style that will add real drama to your look. Pair with sunnies, a bold lip, or earrings for a polished finish.

We used a 28 x 75-inch (70 x 190-cm) scarf to create this look.

Ideally, use a stiff, structured fabric for this style.

Tie hair into a tight topknot.

Place the headscarf at the back of the head, with one of the long edges lowered to the nape of the neck.

Tightly pull the rest of the fabric around to the front, and tie in a knot at the center.

Tie the fabric into a bow (1), hiding the ends within the folds so you're left with a statement, oversized bow (2).

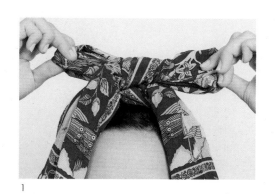

1

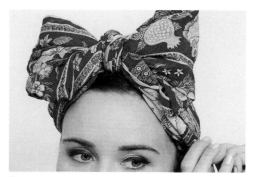

2

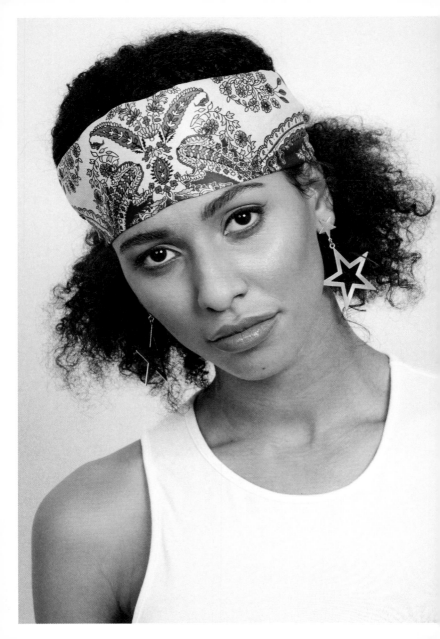

11

The HIPPIE HEADBAND

11: The
HIPPIE
HEADBAND

Channel hippie cool with a retro headband worn with loose tousled waves—great for festivals, beach trips, and vacations.

We used a 35-inch (90-cm) square scarf to create this look.

For this style, it's best to use a silk scarf for its thinness.

Take a square headscarf and fold it into a triangle, then fold again to make a thick band.

With the hair left loose in a center part, wrap the folded scarf around the forehead (1).

Tie tightly, so it doesn't slip, at the back with a knot (2 & 3).

To amplify the hippie vibe, you can work braids into the hair before wrapping the headband.

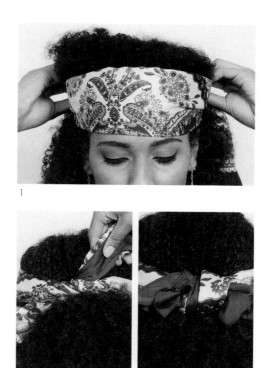

1

2   3

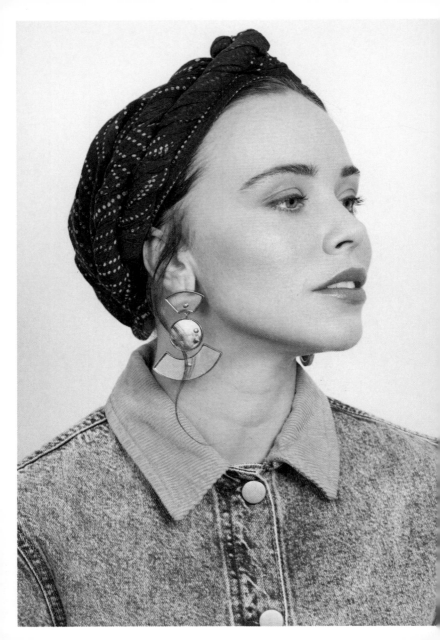

12

The MAIDEN TWIST

12: The MAIDEN TWIST

This pretty, maiden-inspired style will add a unique finish to any outfit, and it looks just as good all year round. Works best with a chiffon or thin cotton scarf.

We used a 20 x 67-inch (50 x 170-cm) scarf to create this look.

Position one edge of a long, rectangular scarf on your forehead, with the fabric draped over the head (1).

Take the ends of the scarf to the back and cross over, trapping the loose fabric underneath so the scarf is in place like a hat (2).

Tightly twist the ends of the fabric to create rope-like strands that you can wrap around the head (3), crossing at the front (4), then tuck them in to secure in place (5).

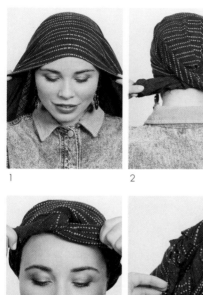

1

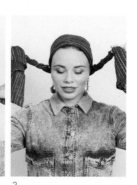

2

3

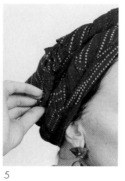

4

5

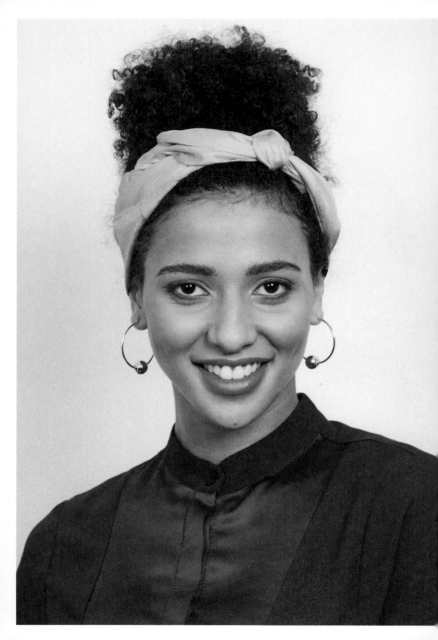

13

The KNOTTED BAND

13: The KNOTTED BAND

Add an elegant, ballerina-inspired finish to your updo with this easy-to-master knotted headband style.

We used a 28-inch (70-cm) square scarf to create this look.

Tie hair into a topknot.

Fold a square scarf into a triangle, then twist until it resembles a long, thin band.

Take to the back of the head and pull the ends of the scarf up to meet at the front (1).

Tie tightly at the top of the head so the band sits securely and comfortably over the ears (2).

Tie a second knot to secure in place (3) and then neaten it up (4).

Tuck the loose ends of the scarf under the band to create a chic and complex-looking wrap (5).

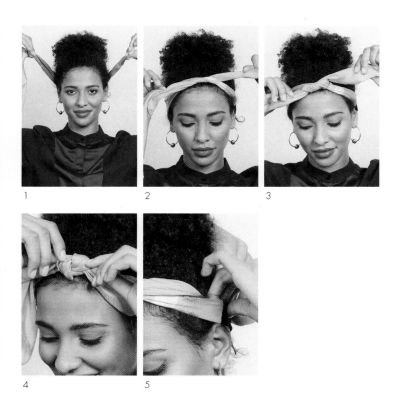

1

2

3

4

5

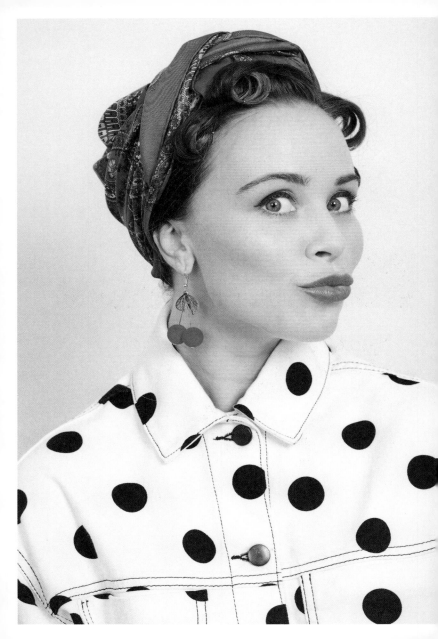

14

The ROLLERS COVER-UP

14: The
ROLLERS
COVER-UP

Keep your rollers covered and neat with the help of a headscarf—a timeless style that's both functional and fashionable.

We used a 28-inch (70-cm) square scarf to create this look.

Take a large, square scarf and fold it into a triangle, then place the fold at the nape of the neck (1).

With the curlers in place, pull the ends of the fabric up over the ears to meet at the top, and tie tightly in a knot, trapping the point underneath so the fabric covers the whole head (2).

Finally, fold the loose triangular point back on itself to conceal the knot (3). Tuck the scarf ends underneath (4).

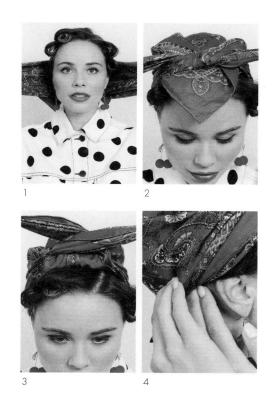

1

2

3

4

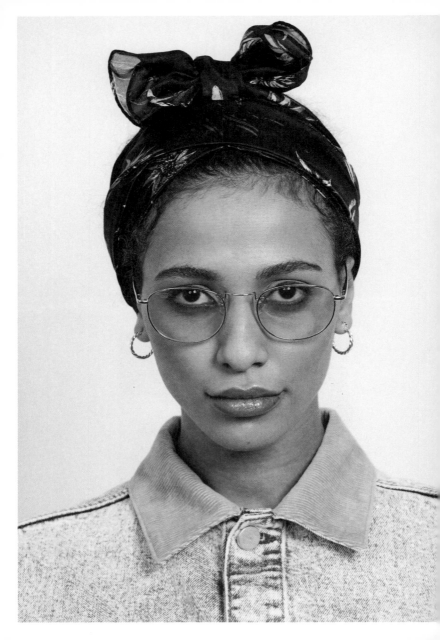

15

The REAR BOW WRAP

15: The
REAR BOW WRAP

Business at the front, party in the back. A ladylike twist on a traditional headwrap that's easy to master but adds instant sass to any look.

We used a 24 x 75-inch (60 x 190-cm) scarf to create this look.

This look works with hair up in a ponytail or down.

Take a large, rectangular scarf (perhaps folded in half lengthwise if a very thin fabric), and put it over the head with one of the long edges along the hairline and the other at the nape of the neck (1).

Draw the ends of the scarf up, to cover the ears and cross over at the top of the head (2).

Bring the ends down to cross again at the base of the head (3), then back up to meet at the top, where you'll just have two short ends of the scarf left.

Cross over and tie the ends of the scarf at the crown of the head into a knot or small bow and use a safety pin to secure in place.

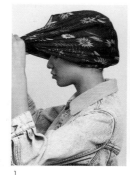

1

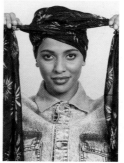

2

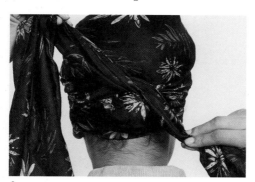

3

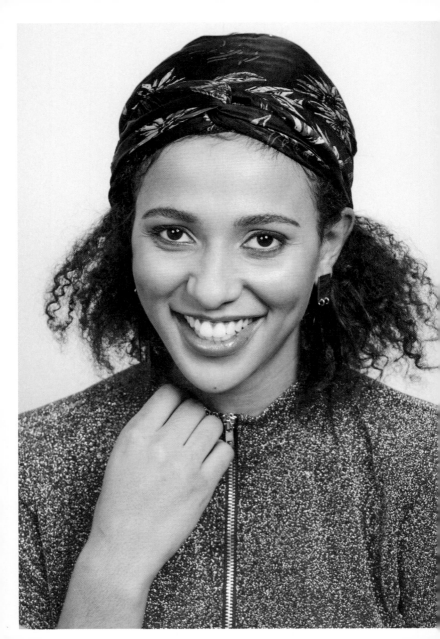

16

The TWISTED WRAP

16: The
TWISTED WRAP

A stylish, statement finish to any outfit that works just as well with the hair up or down. Switch up your scarves with different patterns for different looks.

We used a 24 x 75-inch (60 x 190-cm) scarf to create this look.

With hair down or in a loose, low bun or ponytail, position the scarf over your head with the long edge on your forehead, just below the hairline (1).

Cross the ends of the fabric at the nape of your neck and pull tightly around to the front to meet at the center of the forehead (2).

Twist the ends over each other once or twice, tucking the ends of the fabric underneath the scarf to secure in place (3). If your scarf is very long, knot it at the back first and then tuck the ends under.

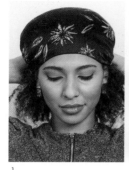

1

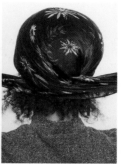

2

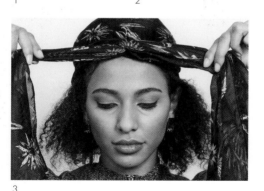

3

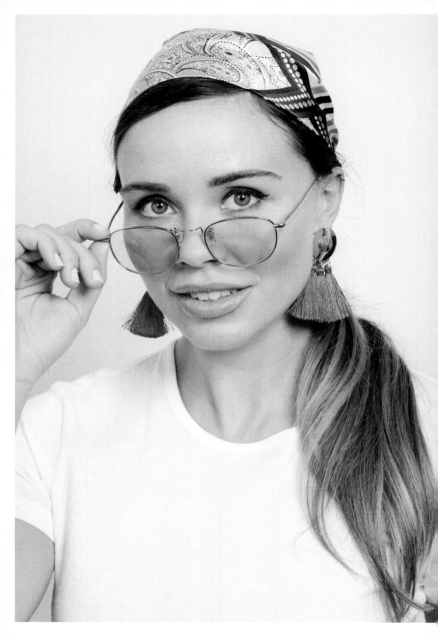

17

The VACATION HEADCOVER

17: The
VACATION HEADCOVER

Say bye-bye to beachy blowaways with this knotted headcover that looks elegant and relaxed, while keeping everything in place.

We used a 24-inch (60-cm) square scarf to create this look.

With hair in a low bun, ponytail, or chignon, fold a square scarf in half to create a triangle.

Take the fold to the top of the forehead (1), leaving your bangs loose if you have them, and draw the ends of the fabric to the back of the head.

Tie the ends in a knot or bow, trapping the point of the triangle underneath to create an elegant covered look (2 & 3).

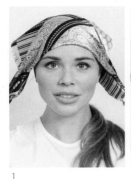
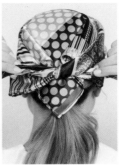

1

2

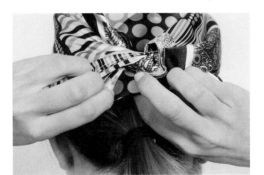

3

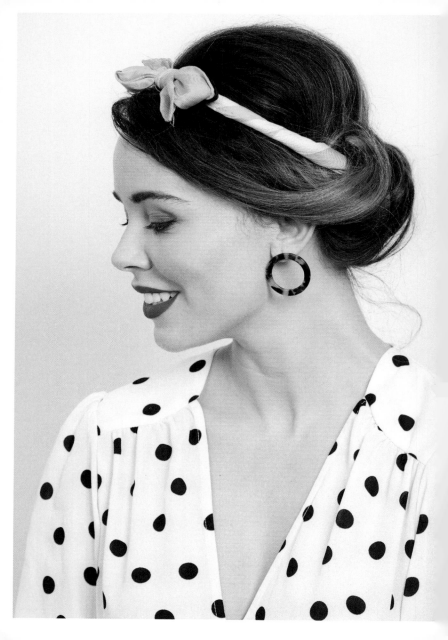

18

The ROLLED UPDO

18: The ROLLED UPDO

A more complex style that works best with longer hair to create an elegant, bohemian look—one to practice, master, and wear to impress.

We used a 28-inch (70-cm) square scarf to create this look.

This style works best with day-old hair or textured hair. Dry shampoo is an easy way to add a bit of instant texture.

Tie hair into an ultraloose ponytail, so that the elastic is toward the lower end of the ponytail.

Take a square scarf and fold it into a triangle, then fold it again to make a band.

Position the scarf over the elastic (1) and roll it toward the base of the head, winding the hair around the scarf as you go (2 & 3).

Pull and position the hair as you roll, so it evenly covers the scarf and sits comfortably at the base of the neck (4).

Bring the two ends to meet at the top of the head (5), then tie in a knot to secure (6).

Loosely pull out some of the hair around the hairline to give a more effortless look. If you have really long hair, you might want to secure the hair roll with pins.

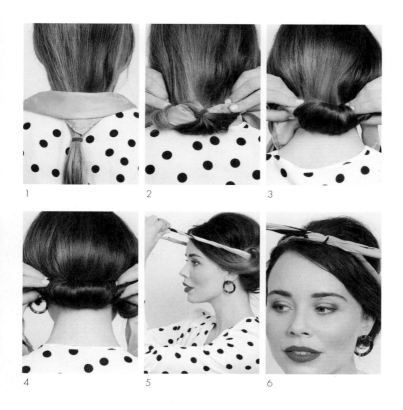

1

2

3

4

5

6

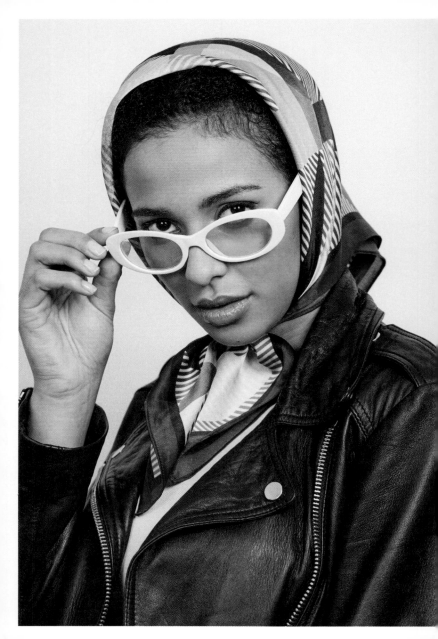

19

The UNDER CHIN TWIST

19: The
UNDER CHIN TWIST

A classic style favored by both Queen Elizabeth II and Audrey Hepburn, this one is timeless, sophisticated, and ladylike. Use different prints for different aesthetics.

We used a 28-inch (70-cm) square scarf to create this look.

Fold a square silk scarf into a triangle and place the fold along the hairline with the point facing down toward the back of the head (1).

Tie the two ends into a single knot under the chin and tighten until the scarf feels comfortable and secure (2).

Once in place, fasten into a double knot (3). You might want to play with the fabric a bit to achieve a more natural look.

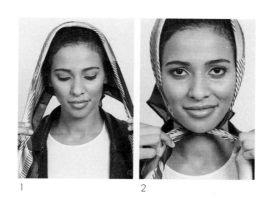

1

2

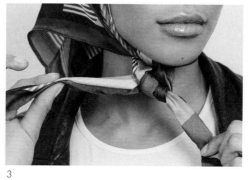

3

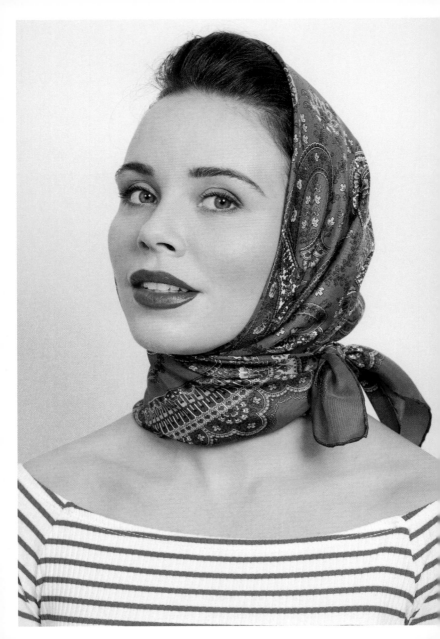

20

The "THELMA & LOUISE" COVER-UP

20: The "THELMA & LOUISE" COVER-UP

Take note from Thelma and Louise with this timeless, sleek, and functional style that keeps everything in place—flyaways, bangs, chignons, the lot.

We used a 35-inch (90-cm) square scarf to create this look.

It's important to use a large enough scarf for this style or you won't have enough fabric.

Fold a large, square scarf into a triangle and place the fold over the head along the hairline with the point facing down your back.

Cross the two ends of the scarf under your chin (1) and wrap around the neck, trapping the point of the scarf (2) so the fabric is pulled tightly and securely over the head.

If the scarf is especially large, tuck in the point at the back after you've secured the knot (3).

Tie the ends in a small knot at the side of the neck to fix in place (4).

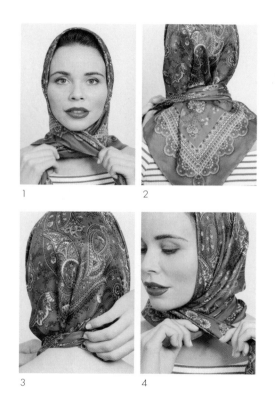

1

2

3

4

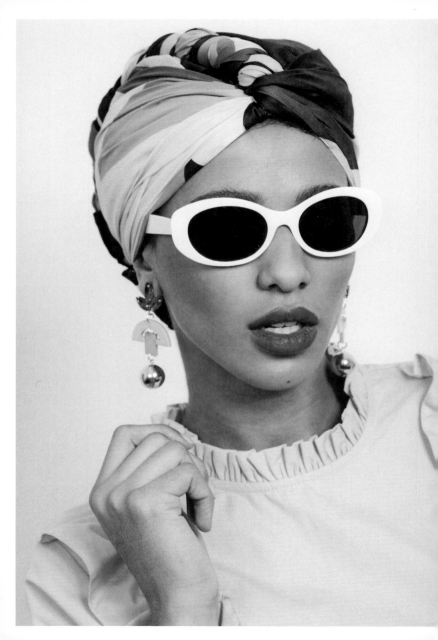

21

The ROPE TWIST COVER-UP

21: The
ROPE TWIST
COVER-UP

This looks great for getting
your hair out of the way
through the summer months.
Get it up, twist, and tuck.
So easy!

We used a 28 x 70-inch
(70 x 180-cm) scarf to create
this look.

Tie hair into a high, tight
ponytail.

Place a long, rectangular
headscarf at the back of
the head, with one of the
long edges at the nape of
your neck (1).

Tightly pull the rest of the
scarf around to the front,
then twist the fabric so that
it sits tightly and securely
around the head (2).

Once fully twisted, take
this "rope" toward the
back of the head and tuck
underneath the scarf at
the nape of your neck to
fasten in place (3–5).

Finish the look with a pair
of statement earrings.

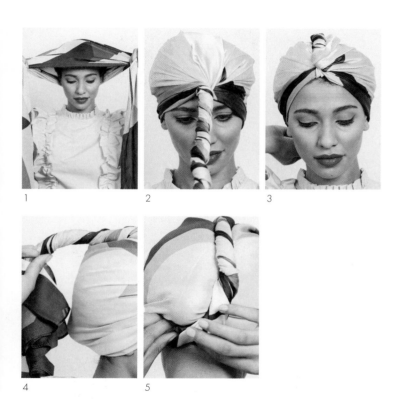

1

2

3

4

5

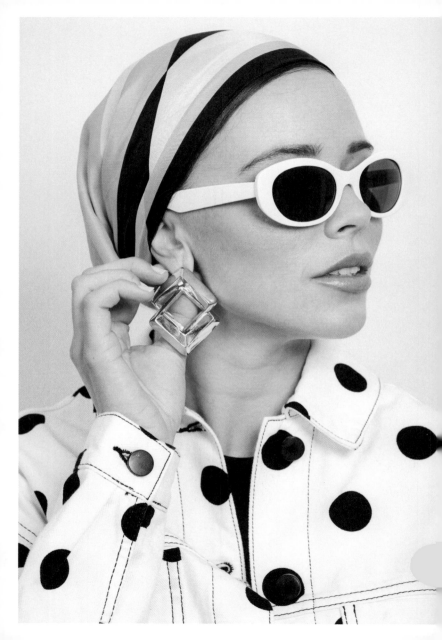

22

The COVERED CHIGNON

22: The
COVERED CHIGNON

A sleek and striking style that's sure to put the finishing touch on any fashion-forward outfit. Best with a printed silk or cotton scarf—and sunnies are a must!

We used a 28-inch (70-cm) square scarf to create this look.

This style works best with the hair tied into a loose chignon.

Fold a square, silk scarf into a triangle and place the fold over the head along the hairline with the point facing down your back (1).

Draw the two ends of the fabric to meet underneath the chignon and fasten in a small knot, tight enough for the scarf to stay securely on your head (2).

Tuck the points of the scarf left over the chignon underneath the knot (3).

Finish the look with statement earrings or a bold lip.

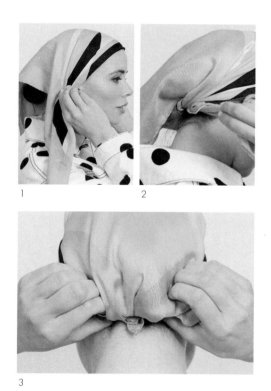

1

2

3

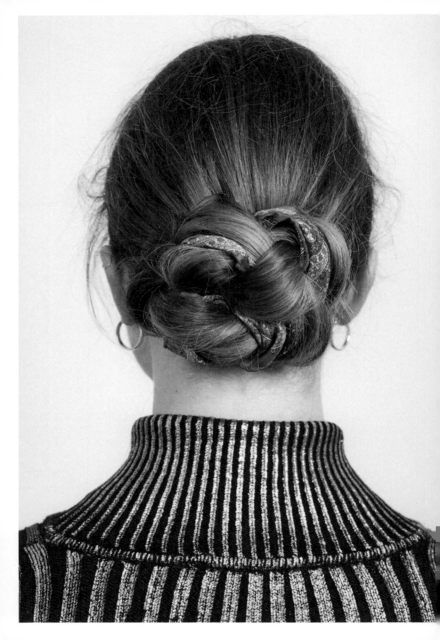

23

The STATEMENT CHIGNON

23: The STATEMENT CHIGNON

Turn a relaxed look into something bright, different, and unexpected by weaving a printed scarf into a loose chignon—a great day-to-night outfit addition!

We used a 20-inch (50-cm) square scarf to create this look.

Tie the hair into a loose, low ponytail.

Take a long, thin scarf and wrap a couple of times around the elastic, so that you end up with equal lengths of the scarf left loose.

Begin to braid the hair, weaving in the scarf ends as you go, and then fasten securely with an elastic band (1).

Loosely wrap the braid into a bun (2) and pin in place to secure (3).

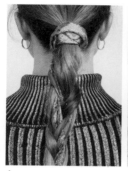

1

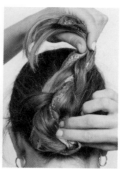

2

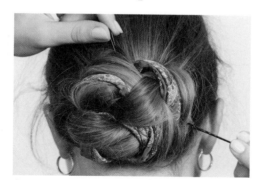

3

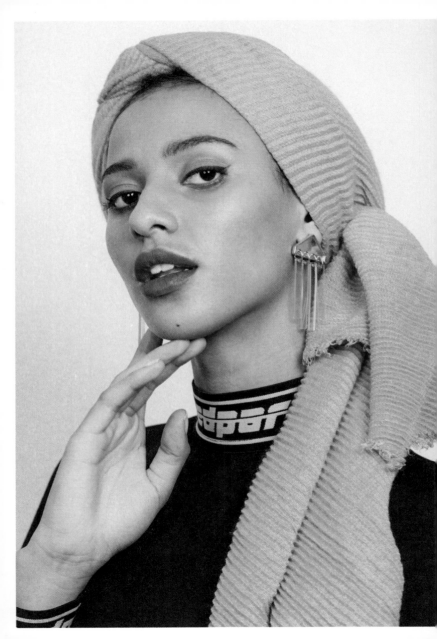

24

The DRAPED WRAP

24: The DRAPED WRAP

Perfect for the winter months and sure to add impact to a laid-back look. Use an oversized scarf for maximum effect!

We used a 28 x 40-inch (70 x 100-cm) scarf to create this look.

The bigger the scarf the better this look works.

With the hair tied in a low bun, take the long edge of a large scarf to the hairline at the front. Bring the ends past the ears to tie, at the nape of your neck (1).

Draw both ends back around to the front and tie again at the top (2).

Take one of the ends directly down, past the ear, and the other, more loosely, over the back of the head and then around to meet at the ear (3). Tie both ends in place here with a secure knot (4).

Leave the remainder of the scarf to drape from this knot over the shoulder, to create a slouchy but statement style.

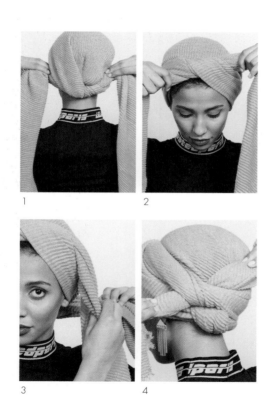

1

2

3

4

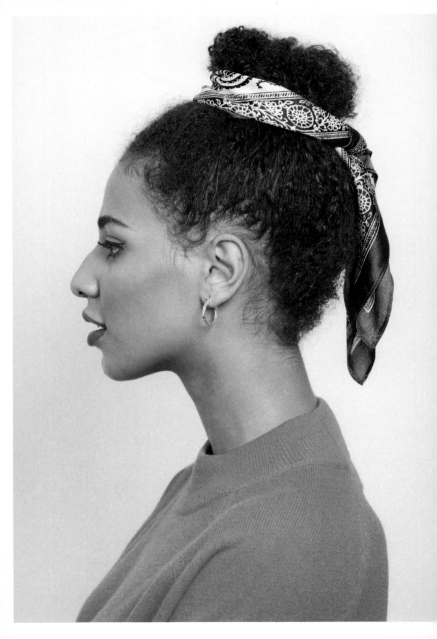

25

The TIED-UP TOPKNOT

25: The
TIED-UP
TOPKNOT

Win the topknot game with the help of a silky square scarf. A foolproof way to make a simple hairstyle impossibly chic.

We used a 20-inch (50-cm) square scarf to create this look.

Tie the hair into a topknot. A hair doughnut is a good way of adding extra volume, and you may need pins to keep everything in place (these can be covered by the scarf).

Once secure, take a small, square silk scarf and fold it into a triangle, then fold again to create a band.

Take this to the base of the topknot at the front (1) and tie tightly with a double knot at the back (2). Leave the scarf ends to hang loose.

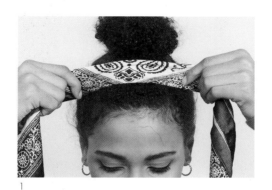

1

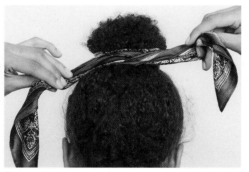

2

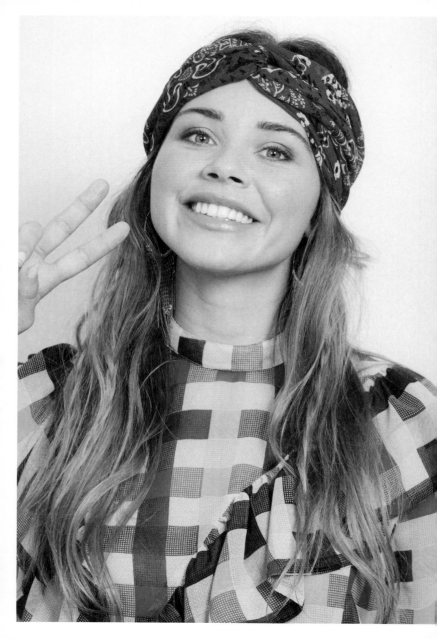

26

The BOHO TWIST

26: The
BOHO TWIST

Turn your loose vacation locks into something more styled with a printed headband. It keeps your hair in place and looks great with loose waves or full braids.

We used a 24 x 75-inch (60 x 190-cm) scarf to create this look.

With the hair left loose in braids (a center part works best for this style), take a long, thin scarf to the back of the head (1) and bring both ends around to cross the forehead.

With a single twist at the front (2), turn each end back on itself to meet at the back.

Before you fasten, take one end under and the other end over the first layer of the band to keep it all together (3), then tie a small double knot (4).

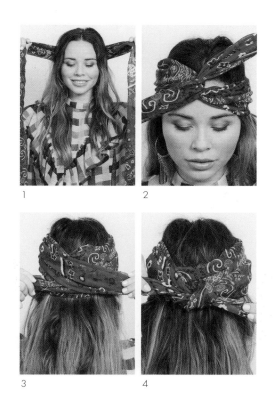

1

2

3

4

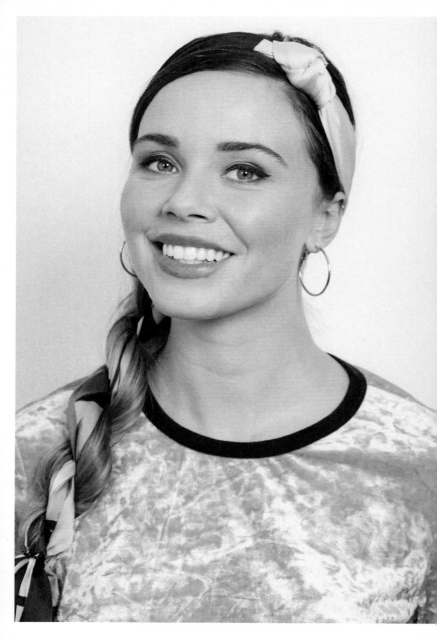

27

The TWISTED BAND

27: The TWISTED BAND

A feminine finish to any outfit that works well with long hair, incorporating both a headband and a braid.

We used a 28 x 70-inch (70 x 180-cm) scarf to create this look.

Start by tying your hair into a loose, low side ponytail. Tie a knot in the center of a long, rectangular scarf (1).

Take the scarf to the top of the head, positioning the knot to one side, and tie under the ponytail so the band feels secure and comfortable (2).

Take the ponytail out so the hair is loose and begin to twist (or braid) the scarf into the hair (3).

When you reach the end, fasten the hair and scarf with an elastic (4).

You might want to play with the twist a bit to loosen it and give it a more relaxed look. You also may want to add pins to the hair around the ears to keep the scarf in place.

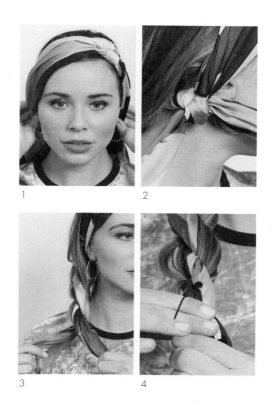

1

2

3

4

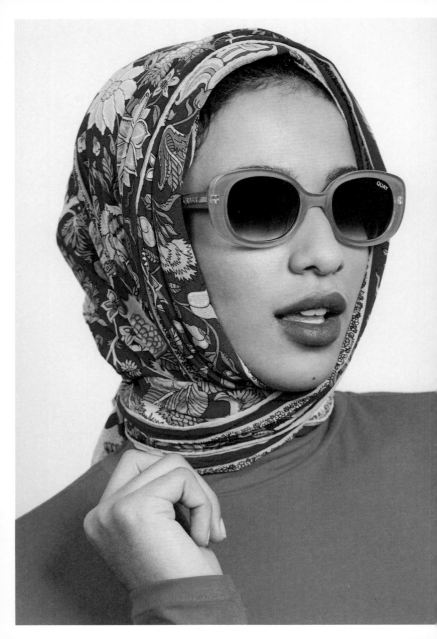

28

The SLOUCHY HEAD WRAP

28: The SLOUCHY HEAD WRAP

A relaxed, slouchy take on a traditional hijab that's easy to create and easy to wear—great for weekends and lazy, low-key days.

We used a 28 x 75-inch (70 x 190-cm) scarf to create this look.

Take a long, rectangular scarf over the head and fasten with a safety pin under the chin (1).

Twist one of the ends of the scarf until it resembles a rope (2), then wrap it around the neck, crossing over the safety pin. Tuck it neatly underneath to secure when you reach the end.

Open out the other end of the scarf so the fabric is wide, then cross this under the chin before wrapping the fabric over the head (3 & 4).

Pin the scarf ends at the back of your head to secure in place (5).

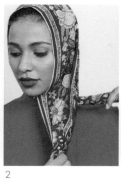

1

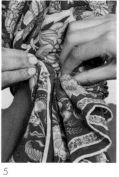

2

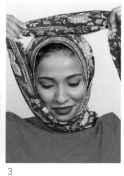

3

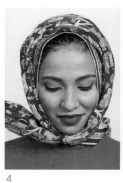

4

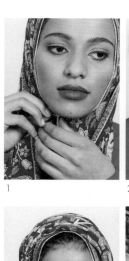

5

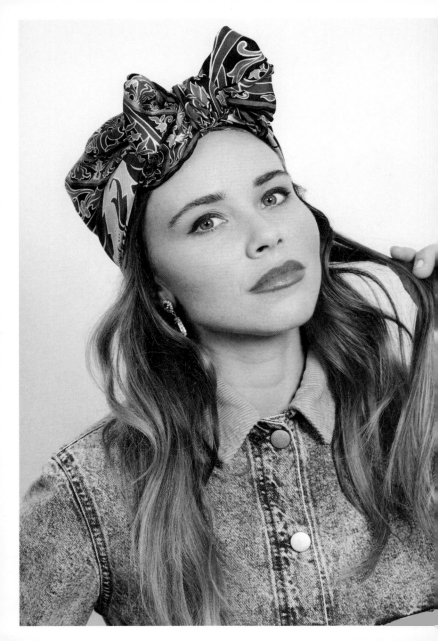

29

The BABY BOW COVER-UP

29: The
BABY BOW
COVER-UP

Add a statement bow to the top of a headwrap to introduce impact and drama to a classic look. This one is a little tricky to master but once you've got it, practice makes perfect!

We used a 35-inch (90-cm) square scarf to create this look.

Fold a large, silk square scarf in half to create a triangle and then place the fold at the nape of the neck (1).

With the point of the triangle facing down over the forehead, bring the other two ends around over the ears and tie tightly at the top of the head (2), trapping the points of the scarf underneath.

Take the point of the triangle over to one side and tuck away neatly under the scarf near the ear (3).

Tie a bow at the front of your head with the two ends of the scarf (4). Tuck the ends of the bow into the headscarf and straighten the bow. Use pins to secure in place, if needed.

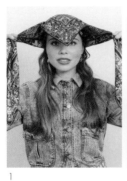

1

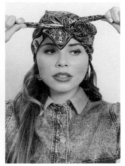

2

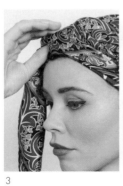

3

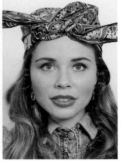

4

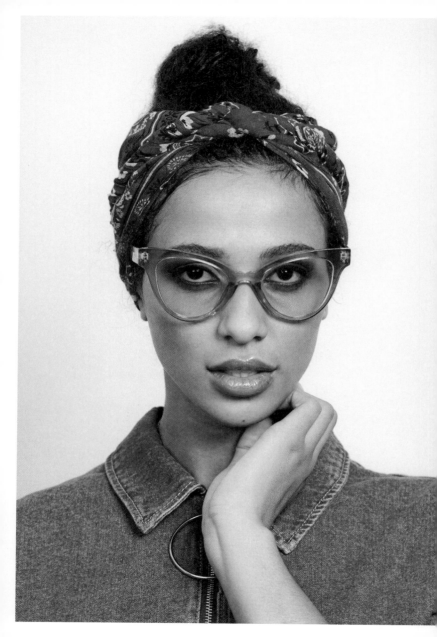

30

The KNOTTED FRONT, BACK, AND SIDES

30: The KNOTTED FRONT, BACK, AND SIDES

A chic style for the colder months (that's great for keeping your ears warm!), this slouchy, knotted style goes well with earrings and a cozy winter coat.

We used a 24 x 75-inch (60 x 190-cm) scarf to create this look.

Fasten the hair into a loose topknot.

Take a long, rectangular scarf to the back of the head (1) and bring the two ends of the fabric to the front.

At the center, cross and then twist them back on themselves (2).

Now twist each end into a rope (3), then fasten in a small knot at the back of the headband (4).

You might want to work with the hair left exposed at the top so it sits nicely within the scarf.

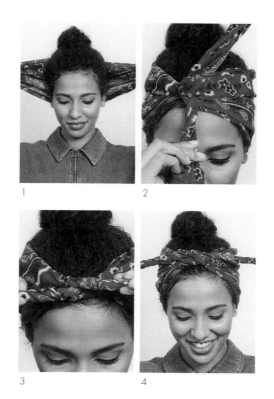

1

2

3

4

About the author

ALICE TATE is a freelance writer and blogger living in London. She studied Fashion Design at the University of Leeds before moving to New York and then Sydney to work for Refinery 29, *W Magazine*, *NYLON*, and *RUSSH*. Alice moved back to the UK to help launch Refinery 29 in London. She also writes for *Grazia*, the *Evening Standard*, The Pool, and *Condé Nast Traveller*. You can also find Alice at her blog, FlashAnthology.com.

Editor: Sarah Massey
Design Manager: Heesang Lee
Production Manager: Sarah Masterson Hally

Library of Congress Control Number:
2018950313

ISBN: 978-1-4197-3725-1

Text copyright © 2018 Pop Press
Photographs copyright © 2018 Pop Press

Cover © 2019 Abrams

First published in the United Kingdom by Ebury, a division of The Random House Group Limited.

Published in 2019 by Abrams Image, an imprint of ABRAMS. All rights reserved. No portion of this book may be reproduced, stored in a retrieval system, or transmitted in any form or by any means, mechanical, electronic, photocopying, recording, or otherwise, without written permission from the publisher.

Printed and bound in China
10 9 8 7 6 5 4 3 2 1

Abrams Image books are available at special discounts when purchased in quantity for premiums and promotions as well as fundraising or educational use. Special editions can also be created to specification. For details, contact specialsales@abramsbooks.com or the address below.

Abrams Image® is a registered trademark of Harry N. Abrams, Inc.

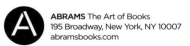

ABRAMS The Art of Books
195 Broadway, New York, NY 10007
abramsbooks.com